Distribution, publication, and copying in any form are prohibited and subject to damages.

TEN HYPNOSES

Copying, publishing, and sharing with third parties are only permitted with the written consent of the author. Please observe the notes on copyright and usage.

Distribution, publication, and copying in any form are prohibited and subject to damages.

Copying, publishing, and sharing with third parties are only permitted with the written consent of the author. Please observe the notes on copyright and usage.

Distribution, publication, and copying in any form are prohibited and subject to damages.

Ingo Michael Simon

TEN HYPNOSES

35
JEALOUSY IN RELATIONSHIPS

Copying, publishing, and sharing with third parties are only permitted with the written consent of the author. Please observe the notes on copyright and usage.

Distribution, publication, and copying in any form are prohibited and subject to damages.

© 2024 Ingo Michael Simon
All rights reserved.
Independently published
www.ingosimon.com

Important Notes for Urgent Attention:

The contents of this book are based on the practical experiences of the author with hypnosis applications and psychotherapy in a trance state. Although the author has strived for the utmost care, errors or misunderstandings in the presentation cannot be completely excluded. Therapeutic work with people and the application of hypnosis are solely the responsibility of the hypnotist. It cannot be ruled out that parts of this book may be misunderstood or that the application of a presented procedure may cause an undesirable reaction in the client. The author also assumes no co-responsibility if work with a client is carried out with reference to the statements in this book.

The Author:

Ingo Michael Simon studied psychology and education and is a hypnotherapist with practices in southwestern Germany and Switzerland. With the help of hypnosis-supported psychotherapy, he primarily treats people with persistent psychological conditions. His practice focuses on anxiety disorders, pathological compulsions, and psychosomatic illnesses. His therapeutic offerings mainly include classical and modern hypnosis applications and the dreamland therapy he developed himself.

Copying, publishing, and sharing with third parties are only permitted with the written consent of the author. Please observe the notes on copyright and usage.

Distribution, publication, and copying in any form are prohibited and subject to damages.

INTRODUCTION — 6

COPYRIGHT AND USAGE — 8

HYPNOSIS 1 — 10

HYPNOSIS 2 — 14

HYPNOSIS 3 — 18

HYPNOSIS 4 — 22

HYPNOSIS 5 — 26

HYPNOSIS 6 — 31

HYPNOSIS 7 — 35

HYPNOSIS 8 — 39

HYPNOSIS 9 — 44

HYPNOSIS 10 — 48

ALL TITLES IN THE SERIES — 53

Copying, publishing, and sharing with third parties are only permitted with the written consent of the author. Please observe the notes on copyright and usage.

Introduction

The series "Ten Hypnoses" is very well known in Germany, Austria, and Switzerland as a collection of texts for therapeutic work and is used by numerous psychotherapeutic practices, doctors, therapists, coaches, and other helping professionals. I am pleased to now be able to offer these texts in other countries as well.

Most therapists have their own methods for inducing and deepening trance as well as for exiting trance. Therefore, I have focused on the main part of the hypnosis. The texts in this book can be integrated as the main part into any hypnosis process. The texts in this collection use various hypnosis techniques. I will not explain these in detail, as I assume that users have the appropriate training. It is also not necessary to understand the exact structure or functioning of the different parts. The texts can simply be read aloud, and they will have their effect.

Decide for yourself which text best suits your client or patient at any given time. You can also combine passages from different texts. It is not about using all ten hypnoses in sequence. It is a selection of possibilities.

I want to emphasize that books cannot replace therapy. Psychotherapy or other therapeutic treatments involve much more. A careful diagnosis is the necessary basis for deciding on the use of methods, including whether hypnosis or one of my texts should be used. Even in this case, preparatory discussions, follow-up discussions during the session, and of course, a therapeutic concept for the sequence of sessions and the content approaches are essential parts of therapy. This cannot and should not be achieved with a collection of texts.

In any case, I wish you much success in your work and I am pleased if my text templates can contribute in a small way.

Ingo Michael Simon

Distribution, publication, and copying in any form are prohibited and subject to damages.

Copyright and Usage

Copying, publishing, and sharing with third parties is prohibited and only permitted with the written consent of the author. Please observe the following copyright and usage guidelines.

This work has been carefully crafted and created to the best of the author's knowledge and personal experience. It comprises text templates and application guidelines for professional hypnosis sessions. The author is a licensed psychotherapist with extensive experience in psychotherapy, coaching, and personal training using hypnotic techniques and methods. Nevertheless, the author and the publisher assume no liability for the accuracy of information, instructions, and advice, nor for any typographical errors. The author and publisher accept no responsibility or liability for the application of these texts and recommendations with clients or patients, nor for any potential consequences or unexpected reactions. It is expressly noted that the application of therapeutic and advisory techniques and formulations lies solely and entirely within the responsibility of the practitioner. This also applies to adherence to the

Copying, publishing, and sharing with third parties are only permitted with the written consent of the author. Please observe the notes on copyright and usage.

boundaries of legally regulated medical and therapeutic practices. The fact that a book containing action proposals is freely available for sale does not imply that its application with clients or patients is permitted for everyone.

Hypnosis 1

… … Today, you can and will let go of the feeling of jealousy and rediscover trust … … because you've realized that this jealousy is completely exaggerated … … … … Today, you can and will let go of the feeling of jealousy and rediscover trust … … because you've decided to be more free and trusting … … … … Today, you can and will let go of the feeling of jealousy and rediscover trust … … because you're allowing all the helpful suggestions to sink deep into your inner being … … … … Today, you can and will let go of the feeling of jealousy and rediscover trust … … because in trance, it's much easier to build and maintain new trust … … … … You can trust … … You can truly trust again … …

… … You know that your mistrust belongs to relationships long past … … and therefore, in your current relationship, you can trust again … … … … You know that your mistrust belongs to relationships long past … … and therefore, you are now truly ready to let go of the past … … … … You know that your mistrust belongs to relationships long past … …

and therefore, you look forward to exploring the present with trust ... ... You know that your mistrust belongs to relationships long past ... ... and therefore, you can truly trust your partner ... ... You can trust ... ... You can truly trust again ... ...

... ... The relaxation of your body helps you feel and remain inwardly calm ... ... and so it becomes easier for you to let go of fear and anxiety again and again ... ... The relaxation of your body helps you feel and remain inwardly calm ... ... and so you can also let go of fearful thoughts and fears of loss ... ... The relaxation of your body helps you feel and remain inwardly calm ... ... and so you can find trust in peace ... ... The relaxation of your body helps you feel and remain inwardly calm ... ... and so the trust within you can grow stronger and stronger ... ... You can trust ... ... You can truly trust again ... ...

... ... Deep in your heart, you feel the love and trust of your partner ... ... and you feel this love for them too ... ... Deep in your heart, you feel the love and trust of your partner ... ... and this love builds more and more trust and closeness ... ...

... ... Deep in your heart, you feel the love and trust of your partner … … and you know that this love is honest and real …

… … Deep in your heart, you feel the love and trust of your partner … … and this love helps you to truly trust … … … … You can trust … … You can truly trust again … …

… … When jealousy arises, you recognize it as an echo from the past that you let fade away … … because by doing so, you free yourself from old and outdated situations … … … … When jealousy arises, you recognize it as an echo from the past that you let fade away … … because by doing so, you overcome past fears and find peace … … … … When jealousy arises, you recognize it as an echo from the past that you let fade away … … because by doing so, you see that the present is completely different … … … … When jealousy arises, you recognize it as an echo from the past that you let fade away … … because by doing so, you experience more and more clearly the loyalty and trust in the present … … … … You can trust … … You can truly trust again … …

… … You feel connected to yourself and now feel a deep sense of calm and relaxation … … and this relaxation accompanies you on your path to trust … … … … You feel connected to yourself and now feel a deep sense of calm and relaxation ... ... and again and again, you find calm and trust in yourself and in your partner ... ... You feel connected to yourself and now feel a deep sense of calm and relaxation ... ... and trust accompanies your journey ... ... trust accompanies your new path ... ... Jealousy fades ... ... You feel connected ... ... You feel truly connected in a trusting relationship ... ...

Hypnosis 2

… … Your goal today is to overcome excessive jealousy and feel free again … … You know that this jealousy is exaggerated and that it stems from past experiences that no longer exist today … … Yet, until now, it hasn't been easy to overcome the jealousy … … Emotions can be powerful, while the mind finds it easier … … In your mind, you probably find it easy to say … … You truly want to let go of the jealousy … … You are using hypnosis to let go of the jealousy deep within … … and when you say it like that, you really mean it … … and that's an important step … … … … In hypnosis, you can hear my words and relax at the same time … … In hypnosis, you are close to your deepest feelings … … You might even say … … Now you feel no jealousy at all … … because you've focused more on the feeling of calm … … That could be the case … … … … Imagine if you could take this experience into your daily life and no longer feel jealousy … … then it would soon become clear … … This hypnosis really ends jealousy… … The suggestions bring you calm and trust … … because only trust can replace jealousy … … That would be brilliant, and maybe it's possible … …

… … Let's imagine for a moment … … You are completely convinced by hypnosis … … and you get to set a goal … … Maybe you would say … … No more jealousy … … because this jealousy bothers you, and you're burdened by it … … … … But your goal could be different, perhaps … … What belongs to the past should stay in the past … … because you know it was relationship breaks and infidelity that made you so jealous … … that could be possible too … … You live in the present … … … … You have thought a lot about jealousy and worked on yourself a lot … … So, it could be that you think … … Jealousy fades as soon as you discover your true feelings … … and that's true … … … … Often, other feelings are behind it … … You can discover and understand them in trance, but maybe you'd rather say … … It's really time to end the jealousy … … and then in the next step … … It's time for the true feelings within you … …

… … You've probably heard someone say … … Deep within, you always find trust … … or … … Deep within, there is no fear or insecurity … … Maybe that's true, and … … deep within lies the solution … … but … … we also live … …

in the everyday world ... ... When you think back, you can probably find a time when it was clear ... ... You trust in honesty and loyalty ... ... because it was also clear ... ... You are absolutely sure that it's worth it ... ... because honesty and loyalty were also shown to you ... ... But then you had different experiences and maybe concluded ... ... Trust is absolutely important to you ... ... but it can also be exploited ... ... But whatever happened before, jealousy and mistrust have caused you pain ... ... At first glance, it seems simple ... ... Trust feels good ... ... Trust brings inner calm ... ... Reaching that again is your goal ... ... I wonder what you would advise a friend who asked for your help to overcome jealousy ... ... Maybe you'd say ... ... You can do this ... ... You can trust ... ... or you might say ... ... Trust yourself, and then trust others ... ...

... ... All the suggestions you've heard now sink deep, and their effects continue to grow ... ... As soon as you notice their effects in your waking life, it becomes clear ... ... Jealousy truly fades ... ... and ... ... Each day, your trust grows stronger and more stable ... ... And when you've experienced that for yourself, and then you meet someone who is also trying to overcome excessive jealousy, you might tell them ... ... Trust yourself... ... because ... ... then you can trust others too ... ... Maybe you'll say to them with complete confidence ... ... You'll see, free from jealousy, you'll feel absolutely great ... ... But wait and observe all the changes you notice in your waking life, critically and closely ... ... Then decide what hypnosis has done for you ... ... You will experience the effect of the suggestions you've heard in your everyday life ... ... and also what has changed there ... ... And as soon as you experience for yourself that jealousy no longer plays a role and you can trust with complete calm again, you have proof and can be sure ... ... This hypnosis truly ended the jealousy ... ... The suggestions you've heard really help you find trust in yourself and in others again and again ... ... Trust in yourself, trust in others ... ... And anyone who uses this hypnosis can experience the same and see for themselves ... ... if ... ... the suggestions take effect ... ...

Hypnosis 3

You are here to overcome jealousy ... ... That is your goal ... ... You want to enjoy your relationship and your life free from fear and with calm ... ... You know that jealousy has grown over time from disappointments and experiences of loss ... ... But these are in the past ... ... You want to be free again ... ... So, let the following suggestions take effect and decide for yourself which ones resonate most with you ... ... Clear suggestions that sound convincing are usually the most powerful ... ... These are the most effective suggestions ... ...

... You truly want to ... let go of jealousy ... [Pause for 5-10 seconds] ... ... You let go of jealousy ... deep within ... [Pause for 5-10 seconds] ... ... This is ... an important step ... [Pause for 5-10 seconds] ... ... Now ... you feel ... no jealousy at all ... [Pause for 5-10 seconds] ... ... The suggestions ... bring you calm and trust ... [Pause for about 30 seconds] ...

... You truly want to ... let go of jealousy ... [Pause for 5-10 seconds] ... ... You let go of jealousy ... deep within ... [Pause for 5-10 seconds] ... ... This is ... an important step ...

[Pause for 5-10 seconds] ... ... Now ... you feel ... no jealousy at all ... [Pause for 5-10 seconds] ... ... The suggestions ... bring you calm and trust ... [Pause for about 30 seconds] ...

... No more ... jealousy ... [Pause for 5-10 seconds] ... ... What belongs to ... the past ... should stay there ... [Pause for 5-10 seconds] ... ... You live ... in the present ... [Pause for 5-10 seconds] ... ... Jealousy fades ... as soon as you ... discover your true feelings ... [Pause for 5-10 seconds] ... ... It is now ... truly time ... for the end of jealousy ... [Pause for 5-10 seconds] ... ... It is time ... for the true feelings ... within you ... [Pause for about 30 seconds] ...

... No more ... jealousy ... [Pause for 5-10 seconds] ... ... What belongs to ... the past ... should stay there ... [Pause for 5-10 seconds] ... ... You live ... in the present ... [Pause for 5-10 seconds] ... ... Jealousy fades ... as soon as you ... discover your true feelings ... [Pause for 5-10 seconds] ... ... It is now ... truly time ... for the end of jealousy ... [Pause for 5-10 seconds] ... ... It is time ... for the true feelings ... within you ... [Pause for about 30 seconds] ...

... Deep within you ... there is always trust ... [Pause for 5-10 seconds] ... ... Deep within lies the solution ... also ... in everyday life ... [Pause for 5-10 seconds] ... ... You trust in ... honesty and loyalty ... [Pause for 5-10 seconds] ... ... You are ... absolutely certain ... that it's worth it ... [Pause for 5-10 seconds] ... ... Trust is ... absolutely important to you ... [Pause for 5-10 seconds] ... ... Trust ... feels good ... [Pause for 5-10 seconds] ... ... You can do this ... ... You can trust ... [Pause for about 30 seconds] ...

... Deep within you ... there is always trust ... [Pause for 5-10 seconds] ... ... Deep within lies the solution ... also ... in everyday life ... [Pause for 5-10 seconds] ... ... You trust in ... honesty and loyalty ... [Pause for 5-10 seconds] ... ... You are ... absolutely certain ... that it's worth it ... [Pause for 5-10 seconds] ... ... Trust is ... absolutely important to you ... [Pause for 5-10 seconds] ... ... Trust ... feels good ... [Pause for 5-10 seconds] ... ... You can do this ... ... You can trust ... [Pause for about 30 seconds] ...

... Each day ... your trust grows stronger and more stable ... [Pause for 5-10 seconds] ... ... Free from jealousy ... you feel absolutely great ... [Pause for 5-10 seconds] ... ... The suggestions ... you've heard help you ... always find trust ... [Pause for 5-10 seconds] ... ... Trust ... in yourself ... trust ...

also in others ... [Pause for 5-10 seconds] ... ... The ... suggestions take effect ... [Pause for about 30 seconds] ...

... Each day ... your trust grows stronger and more stable ... [Pause for 5-10 seconds] ... ... Free from jealousy ... you feel absolutely great ... [Pause for 5-10 seconds] ... ... The suggestions ... you've heard help you ... always find trust ... [Pause for 5-10 seconds] ... ... Trust ... in yourself ... trust ... also in others ... [Pause for 5-10 seconds] ... ... The ... suggestions take effect ... [Pause for about 30 seconds] ...

Hypnosis 4

... ... You embrace today's hypnosis with joy and trust ... ... because this allows you to let go of the fear of being abandoned today and find new trust ... ...

... ... You are determined to absorb all the suggestions deep within yourself ... ... because this allows you to let go of the fear of being abandoned today and find new trust ... ...

... ... You are ready to allow the suggestions to take full effect now ... ... because this allows you to let go of the fear of being abandoned today and find new trust ... ...

... ... Today, you are embarking on a new path, your new path ... ... because this allows you to let go of the fear of being abandoned today and find new trust ... ...

... ... You know that part of your fear of being abandoned exists only in your thoughts ... ... and that's why you can truly let go of fears and worries ... ... You know that your thoughts can influence your feelings ... ... and that's why you can truly let go of fears and worries ... ... You know that thoughts can even strengthen our intentions and goals ... ... and that's why you can truly let go of fears and worries ... ... You know that disturbing thoughts can be let go and replaced with new ones ... ... and that's why you can truly let go of fears and worries ... ... You trust in the help of your subconscious and let go ... ...

... ... Your body has stored every feeling for you and can make it available to you at any time ... ... and that's why you can now feel self-confidence and self-assurance again ... ...

... ... Your body can adopt a strong and confident posture and is already doing so ... ... and that's why you can now feel self-confidence and self-assurance again ... ... Your body helps you to project a confident and secure presence ... ... and that's why you can now feel self-confidence and self-assurance again ... ... Your body willingly takes on a secure and strong posture for you ... ... and that's why you can now feel self-confidence and self-assurance again ... ... You trust in the help of your subconscious and let go ... ...

... ... In trance, you feel particularly connected to yourself and at peace ... ... and that's why you know that you will never lose yourself ... ... You remember that you have always been a reliable partner to yourself ... ... and that's why you know that you will never lose yourself ... ...

You know that your fear is an expression of the deep need for support within yourself ... ... and that's why you know that you will never lose yourself ... ... You find deep trust and support within yourself, always and at all times ... ... and that's why you know that you will never lose yourself ... ... You trust in the help of your subconscious and let go ... ...

... ... You overcome your insecurity and worry with confidence and trust that you now find within yourself ... ... and in doing so, you let go of all fear and find deep trust within yourself ... ... You end jealousy and control because they were only holding you back ... ... and in doing so, you let go of all fear and find deep trust within yourself ... ... You go through the day with trust and courage, focusing on the beauty around you ... ... and in doing so, you let go of all fear and find deep trust within yourself ... ... You approach others with trust and openness, especially in your relationship ... ... and in doing so, you let go of all fear and find deep trust within yourself ... ... You trust in the help of your subconscious and let go ... ...

... ... The suggestions you've heard take root deeper and deeper ... ... and that's why you truly let go of fear and turn again and again to trust and calm ... ... All the suggestions flow deep into your subconscious and stay there ... ... and that's why you truly let go of fear and turn again and again to trust and calm ... ... As soon as you are fully awake again, the suggestions you've heard will become even stronger ... ... and that's why you truly let go of fear and turn again and again to trust and calm ... ... You are free from fear ... ... You are filled with trust ... ... You are truly free from fear ... ... You are truly filled with trust ... ...

Hypnosis 5

… … You've realized that jealousy is a result of an old, outdated fear … … fear of losing someone you care about … … You've decided to let go of this old fear because you want to be free again … … and because you'd much rather experience your life and especially your relationship with trust and calm … … You're here today to achieve just that … … and so you are open to following an inner vision … … because you know that thoughts create inner images when you imagine something … … Maybe you also know that inner images create new feelings … … and new truths … …

That's what you need … … a new truth within you … … the truth of trust … … You don't have to do anything special … … You just need to be here and open yourself to the words you hear … … Let all the words you hear become thoughts and images … …

… … Jealousy is like a sudden storm … … like gray clouds that can suddenly break loose inside you and produce an incredibly strong and furious storm … … With this very image, you can free yourself from jealousy today … …

Imagine these gray clouds within you ... ... in your subconscious ... ... There is a gray cloud of fear ... ... fear of losing someone you care about ... ... Look at the image of this gray cloud before your inner eye, because by doing so, you also recognize this feeling within you ... ... an old feeling that has nothing to do with today's time ... ... With the image of the gray cloud comes the old feeling back and becomes clear ... ... the feeling of fear ... ... fear of losing someone ... ...

You've probably already lost people who were important to you ... ... maybe even someone very special ... ... and the fear has remained until today ... ... But today is the day when the old fear should go because that time is over ... ... Nothing ever happens twice in life, and every stage of life contains new chances and opportunities ... ... The gray cloud of past fear of loss is like a thick rain cloud from which the storms of jealousy could break forth ... ... But that changes today ... ... But that changes now ... ... And before your inner eye, this cloud begins to rain ... ... like ancient tears, the fear rains out of the gray cloud ... ... It rains and rains ... ...

Tears rain down to the ground ... ... more and more ... ... The past fear now finds its way as a feeling of sadness and mourning ... ... You know what made you so sad, you feel it again now ... ... You know that this sadness and the fear of experiencing it again produced the jealousy ... ... But the old tears are dissolving ... ... and the old fear is fading ... ... It becomes lighter inside you ... ... With every raindrop, with every tear, you become freer ... ... [Here, please remain silent for about 20 seconds] ... ...

And the cloud becomes brighter ... ... It becomes brighter and brighter because the old fear finds its way into memory, where it belongs ... ... As a memory, the painful time will remain, but you are freed from the gray cloud of tears and fear ... ... Like a white summer cloud, it drifts further across the sky ... ... [Here, please remain silent for about 20 seconds] ... ...

Now it's time to build new trust ... ... that's easy now because the disturbing cloud of fear is gone ... ... and with it the disturbing feeling of fear ... ... Now you are free for something new ... ... Now you are open for something new ... ... Now you are ready for something new ... ... ready for new trust ... ... And suddenly it's like an inner sunrise ... ... like a shining sun that suddenly rises on the horizon after the rain ... ... and with the image of a rising sun within you, new trust is born ... ... You see the rising sun of trust before your inner eye ... ... a sun that rises higher and higher, and with it the rising feeling of trust ... ... trust in yourself ... ... trust in the help of your subconscious ... ... trust in the effect of hypnosis ... ... trust in your partner ... ... real trust ... ... real trust ... ... The sun rises higher and becomes brighter ... ... It shines stronger and stronger ... ... and the feeling of trust grows stronger within you ... ... so strong that you can feel it more and more clearly ... ... You can trust ... ... You want to trust ... ... You trust ... ... Yes, you trust ... ...

[Here, please remain silent for about 20 seconds] ... ...

This new trust in yourself and in life accompanies you every day from now on ... ... even and especially when you are awake again and go about your daily life ... ... Especially in your everyday life, you can best see that the old feelings of fear keep disappearing, like rain sinking into the ground ... ... and again and again, you feel the inner sun of trust rise ... ... Just as you can imagine it as an image today, so it happens in your feelings every day anew ... ... Maybe you're already wondering when you'll feel and recognize it clearly for the first time in your waking life ... ... Yes, the jealousy is over ... ... Yes, trust is back ... ... Yes, trust feels good ... ...

Hypnosis 6

You have dealt with your jealousy and have recognized that it stands in your way ... ... You've already understood that jealousy finds no justification in the present but stems from past experiences in your life ... ... It arose in the past, and you want to return it to the past ... ... Today, you can talk to an entity that can really help you overcome jealousy ... ... Maybe you are religious and can pray ... ... to God or to Jesus or to an angel ... ... or you talk to yourself because you believe there is a power deep within you that can and will help you ... ... your subconscious or your reflection ... ... Decide for yourself whom you want to talk to, but you always speak with an important and strong part of yourself ... ... with a part that listens to you and supports you ... ... You might say ... ...

Dear Self in the Mirror / Dear God / Dear Guardian Angel / Dear Subconscious ... ... I understand that I must overcome my jealousy ... ... I know that it is inner fears that lead me to be jealous and to suspect without cause that my partner might be unfaithful ... ... I know that my fear and distrust were not caused by them but by past experiences ... ... by past relationships that are already gone ... ... and so it should be ... ... Dear Self in the Mirror / Dear God / Dear Guardian Angel / Dear Subconscious ... ... I ask for your help so that I can truly hand over the past to the past and always remind myself that my relationship today has nothing to do with the past ... ... because only then will I truly be free from jealousy ... ... and I want to be free ... ... I truly want to be free ... ...

Dear Self in the Mirror / Dear God / Dear Guardian Angel / Dear Subconscious ... ... I am fully aware that I need to find and give trust again ... ... Only with trust can a happy and contented relationship succeed ... ... I trust in your guidance and help ... ... Yes, I trust that you ... ... dear Self in the Mirror / dear God / dear Guardian Angel / dear Subconscious ... ... can and want to help me ... ... and I also want to do my part and really try and make an effort ... ... I am fully aware that it requires my strong will to give trust again, but I can do it ... ... I am sure I can do it and that with your support, I will truly succeed ... ... I want that ... ... I truly want to trust ... ... I truly want to be calm and free from fear ... ... I truly want to be fair because I know that my partner is faithful and that my distrust only comes from my past experiences ... ...

Dear Self in the Mirror / Dear God / Dear Guardian Angel / Dear Subconscious ... ... I know that I must first overcome my fear ... ... my fear of being betrayed or abandoned ... ... I am ready for it ... ... With your help and support ... ... dear Self in the Mirror / dear God / dear Guardian Angel / dear Subconscious ... ... I will achieve it ... ... I also know that I need to take care of all my feelings ... ... I want and will accept all my feelings and recognize them as my own ... ... feelings that no one is responsible for and no one brings about guiltily ... ... They arise within me, and I know that my feelings help me, even those that feel painful or unclear ... ... What is important is to accept my feelings as my inner experience, and I want to do that with your help ... ... dear Self in the Mirror / dear God / dear Guardian Angel / dear Subconscious ... ... from today on, again and again ... ...

Dear Self in the Mirror / Dear God / Dear Guardian Angel / Dear Subconscious ... ... Please also help me to stay strong if I do become jealous again ... ... that I continue to believe that I can let go and overcome this feeling ... ... especially when I feel it again ... ... I know I also need to be patient with myself ... ... Maybe my inner self needs some time to fully overcome the jealousy ... ... then I want to give myself that time ... ... I thank you now for your support ... ... dear Self in the Mirror / dear God / dear Guardian Angel / dear Subconscious ... ...

Good ... ... Allow yourself now to enjoy the calm a little longer and simply be here because now you don't have to do anything else ... ... Everything important has already been done ... ... Now the support of your helper becomes the support within you ... ... the help from you for you ... ... So you can rely on double help ... ... So your deepest inner self prepares to do everything that helps you overcome and finally let go of jealousy and build new trust ... ... Trust that you can give again ... ... your trust ... ... your true trust ... ...

Hypnosis 7

… … You want to overcome jealousy today … … You want to be free again and be able to focus on love, affection, and trust … … You want to live and experience your relationship calmly and with a sense of security … … Closeness and connection to yourself are the starting point for constructive and trusting relationships with others … … So today, you find the way to yourself and, with that, the way to trust … …

Your subconscious helps you with this because it hears and understands my words, which become your own words if you want them to … … and you want to overcome jealousy … … that's why you also want to hear and accept the helpful words … … You say them inwardly with me … … You make them your words to free yourself today … … You make them your words to also free your partner from jealousy … … So you are the one who says … …

… … I look deep within myself because I recognize all my feelings there, and because it is easier for me to see with an inward gaze that jealousy only arose within me … … and my deepest inner self reveals all my feelings, even the beautiful and trusting ones ... ...

... ... I look even deeper within myself to find feelings of trust and security there again, to activate my self-confidence ... ... and trustfully and gently, my deepest inner self catches me with a gentle hand ... ...

... ... With curiosity and enthusiasm, I encounter myself in the depths of my feelings to understand myself better and to end my jealousy ... ... and my deepest inner self, this special part of me, meets me halfway with the same curiosity and joy ... ...

... ... I am truly ready to meet myself and my feelings and, with that, the feeling of jealousy to find trust again behind it ... ... and with that, my fellow human beings also come to me with trust and openness ... ...

... ... I accept myself with all my facets and strive for constructive development towards true trust ... ... and more and more, I experience that others also meet me with honest trust ... ...

... ... I trust myself, and I know that this trust helps me let go of fear of loss and mistrust to build new trust ... ... and I experience that stronger trust and more respect are shown to me by others ... ...

... ... What I give myself returns to me as a gift ... ...

... ... I look forward to being able to genuinely trust my partner again and openly give my trust ... ... and I also enjoy the real and honest trust of my partner in me ... ...

... ... I admit and openly express it when I recognize fear of loss and feel jealousy, and I accept them as my feelings ... ... and free from the burden of mistrust, I experience the honest and considerate support given to me from outside ... ...

... ... I trust my partner and my fellow human beings because I feel who is sincere, and because trust is a gain for me ... ... and full of trust and honesty, my fellow human beings approach me and are pleased with my constructive development ... ...

... ... I feel deep within me that with my inward gaze, I have found trusting and constructive thoughts again ... ... and I experience trust every day in my encounters with others ... ...

… … I recognize again and again that jealousy, insecurity, and mistrust only belong to me and have nothing to do with my fellow human beings in the present … … and every day, I experience affection from people who are finally freed and relieved … …

… … In my special development, I am an enrichment for the world because I am unique and constantly evolving … … and I experience my fellow human beings as an enrichment for my own life because I also value their uniqueness and accept it … …

Hypnosis 8

… … You are fighting against jealousy … … You don't want to be jealous yourself, and your mind keeps telling you that everything is fine … … You know that your mistrust comes from your own, especially from past experiences … … Your mind trusts … … and in a state of calm, you can always see clearly that your suddenly arising jealousy … … your sudden fear of betrayal … … fear of being betrayed … … is exaggerated … … You might even say it yourself … … unfair … … because you know that the jealousy doesn't come from your current relationship … … that it has nothing to do with it … … So you absolutely want and as quickly as possible to let go of jealousy … …

… … Jealousy is like a helpless and fearful attempt to hold on … … and you've experienced that with this excessive jealousy, you're more likely to drive a person away from you … … But now you're here to find help … … Now you're here to take a new path … … Now you're here to find the feeling of deep and warm trust again … … because one thing is certain … … Where there is trust, there can be no jealousy …

... You've chosen trust, so it's mainly about feeling that feeling again ... ... and being sure ... ... Yes, you trust ... ... That's what matters ... ... So now I will help you find the feeling of warm and warming trust again ... ... All the feelings we have show up in our body ... ...

... ... Now feel your body ... ... Become aware of your body feeling now ... ... There is, for example, relaxation ... ... Your muscles are relaxed ... ... Your breathing is calm and even ... ... That corresponds to the feeling of calm and tranquility ... ... It's easy to be calm now because you are in a pleasant trance ... ... It's easy to be relaxed now because you are in a pleasant trance ... ...

... ... It's easy to feel any feeling that is there now because you are in a pleasant trance ... ... Trust is also there now because trust is always within you ... ... You always trust in something ... ... maybe in a special ability you have ... ... Maybe you feel this trust and just feel it ... ... or you find it in your body feeling because it's definitely there ... ...

... ... Trust lies in the center of the body, in the inner center ... ... in your stomach ... ... Maybe you're thinking now that mistrust also lies there ... ... in the gut feeling ... ...

Mistrust feels cramped and tense ... ... Trust feels warm and warming ... ... Now place your hand on your stomach, just below your breastbone, so that you don't feel any bones or ribs when you press lightly with your hand on your stomach ... ... good ... ... That's where warm and warming trust sits ... ... warm trust for you ... ... warm self-trust ... ... and warming trust from you for others ... ... Trust in your relationship ... ... Trust and loyalty ... ... Trust in the ability to trust ... ...

... ... Feel the warmth between your palm and your stomach ... ... With a very light pressure of your hand, you can feel the warmth of your body even more clearly because the feeling of trust also becomes clearer ... ... Trust lies as warmth in your body ... ... right where your hand lies ... ... and from there, the warmth flows into your entire body and strengthens the feeling of trust ... ... Trust from you for you ... ... Trust from you for others ... ... Let the warm and warming feeling become clear ... ...

... ... You feel it as actual warmth between your hand and your stomach ... ... and just as real as the warmth is the feeling of trust and the ability to trust, which grows bigger and bigger ... ... From this warm and warming spot, warmth now flows into and through your entire body ... ... and with it, the feeling of trust permeates you more and more … … Warmth flows everywhere … … into every corner of your body … … Trust flows everywhere … … into every corner of your body … … Every cell in your body is informed about warmth and trust … … Every cell trusts … … Every single cell in your body trusts … … And you radiate this trust outward … … Feel the warmth more and more clearly … …

… … Feel the warmth and allow it to flow through your entire body more and more … … as a pleasant warmth … … as a pleasant feeling … … as a feeling of trust … … From your inner center, warmth flows into and through your entire body … … and trust spreads … … Trust spreads within you … … You feel it … … You feel the trust, and you know that jealousy completely dissolves in it … … Trust spreads more and more clearly … … This is the end of jealousy … …

… … Continue to breathe calmly and evenly and trust that with each further breath, your body spreads more inner warmth … … and more trust … … Trust that with each further breath, jealousy disappears if it could even still be there … … Jealousy is over … … It fades away again and again because now is the time of trust … …

… … Now is the time of warm and warming trust … … Now begins a new time … … Now begins a new life … … a life full of trust … … your life full of trust … … your life full of trust … …

Hypnosis 9

… … You want to overcome jealousy today … … you want to free yourself from fear and insecurity … … you want to free yourself from sudden anger … … You've made a really good decision because none of this has anything to do with jealousy … … It's a fake feeling … … Jealousy was created once, but it only covered up an old fear and tried to avoid losses … … Today, you take a journey through time to the starting point, and maybe you're already wondering where the jealousy actually comes from and are quite curious … … or you're just glad that on an inner journey through time, you can let go of jealousy … … Once you learned to find security in jealousy, today you learn to be completely safe without jealousy … …

… … In your feeling, you are taking a journey through space and time … … to find a time when there was no jealousy yet … … to find a time when trust was completely natural … … Maybe you can remember that time … … You were much freer then because trust was completely normal for you … … But it might also seem to you as if jealousy has always been there, but that's not true ... ... But it might have been a very long time since you could really trust ... ... maybe you could only do that as a very small child, who knows ... ... So it could be a short journey or a very long journey into the past, but there was that time when trust was still there ... ... This journey is easy, it goes on its own because your subconscious knows this time of trust and finds it for you ... ... You don't have to do anything special for it, you don't need to have a memory in your thoughts ... ... Just imagine that you are going inward to the time before jealousy ... ... to a time when there were still feelings of trust and security in you ... ... so much trust and so much security that you can feel these feelings now ... ... You feel safe now, in this pleasant trance ... ... You are in trust, enjoy the feeling of trust ... ... [Stay silent for about 20 seconds] ... ...

... ... And now the inner journey continues, and with you travels your trust ... ... With trust and in security, your journey through time continues ... ... You start in the trusting past and slowly move towards the time of jealousy ... ... to find the day when jealousy began ... ... You remember events in your life on this journey ... ... You are approaching a special event ... ... It shook you ... ... maybe a loss or a disappointment ... ... maybe a betrayal or deceit ... ... Something happened that unsettled you ... ... With your trust in your luggage, you approach this day ... ... this event that unsettled you so much ... ... Maybe there were many events that could damage your trust ... ... maybe there were also a few special ones ... ... or maybe it was one very special event that could shape you so much ... ... You find it now ... ... But even if you don't have a clear memory of it now, you are there ... ... You are there now, and a part of you remembers that this is where jealousy arose ... ... You are there, and you recognize what changed you so much ... ...

... ... If you have vivid memories, look at them because you feel good now, and you feel trust ... ... If you don't recognize any images, just feel deep into your feeling because it is the feeling of that time ... ... but it felt different than jealousy ... ... It was a different feeling that was in you ... ... maybe the feeling of being alone or being overlooked ... ... maybe of being abandoned or not finding anyone to turn to in your inner distress and fear ... ... Maybe you needed protection, but there was no one there who could protect or wanted to protect you ... ... There was sadness in you ... ... You now change your attitude towards the events back then

...... You free yourself from jealousy ...... You now know that it was always about very different feelings ...... So you now reactivate the earlier feelings of trust and self-confidence ...... In the calm you feel now, you also find trust in yourself and trust in others ...... The new feeling of the past ...... because trust gets you through any sad time safely ...... and trust becomes the new feeling of today's time ...... Sadness fades ...... Trust remains ...... [Stay silent for about 20 seconds] ......

...... With the feeling of trust, you now slowly return, and on the return journey, you go through your entire lifetime in a few seconds since then, but now trust accompanies you through your life, deep trust ...... Jealousy can no longer arise ...... You now go through the time of your life and learn new and different things than you did back then ...... You now learn to preserve the new feeling of trust and security when you arrive in the present ...... trust in the present, real trust ...... You return to the present ......

Hypnosis 10

... ... There is a special place deep within you ... ... a place of creativity and imagination ... ... a place where memories live and wait for you so that you can always learn from your own experience ... ... This place is the land of dreams ... ... The dreams there are like night dreams with surprises and with images that simply appear ... ... because feelings are suddenly there and show themselves ... ... Maybe you know that the images of night dreams are actually feelings ... ... So it is here ... ... But the land of dreams is also like daydreams ... ... like daydreams in which you can create new images and decide for yourself what direction your dream will take ... ... So imagine being there ... ... deep in your feelings ... ... deep in your imagination ... ... deep in the land of dreams ... ...

... ... You stand at an iron fence that runs through the land of dreams ... ... It seems to divide it into two halves ... ... The fence is so high that you can't climb over it, and you can't find a gate or passage ... ... So you walk along the fence, along this border ... ... You hear noises and can perceive voices that you know ... ... You heard them once in the past ... ... and beyond the fence, you see an event from your past ... ... It was a separation ... ... You had to part from someone, or this person parted from you, left ... ... You see this person on the other side and see again how it was ... ... Like a play from a long-past time, you can watch it here, separated by the high and massive fence ... ... That's how it felt back then too ... ... like an inner fence ... ... There was no getting through ... ... You couldn't stop this person, you just had to accept the separation, maybe even the sudden separation ... ...

... ... That was hard because you didn't want it that way ... ... Back then, there was no other choice for you; you couldn't decide whether you wanted to keep this person in your life ... ... It wasn't your decision, but it was reality ... ... It was suddenly like this fence that you can't just climb over ... ... You couldn't do anything to change the situation ... ... So now you walk close to the fence ... ... Maybe you want to call out something to this person today ... ... But it is a picture of a past time ... ...

... ... The past doesn't change today either, because it never does ... ... As hard as it is to accept, no moment happens twice … … What you see is part of your life story … … The land of dreams wants to help you accept this life story as it was … … You don't have another one … … … … So you keep walking along the fence … … What lies beyond the fence and thus in the past, you can look at but no longer change … … Then you discover a person on the other side who stands with their back to you on a riverbank … … You hear the water rushing … … It is the river of life that always flows on … … just as life moves forward relentlessly … … and although the river seems unchanged as you look at it, it changes every second … … If you imagine the path of a drop of water in the river like the second of a life, then you easily recognize that this drop flows by and will never be in the same place twice … …

… … While the river seems to change little, just as life sometimes seems to stand still and show no more changes, the one drop flows steadily onward … … The person on the riverbank turns around … … You recognize who it is because you look into your own face … … You yourself stand there on the other side of the fence … … But at the same time, you stand here and can't get through the fence, you can't reach yourself … … Jealousy has taken over your life … …

This is how it was created in the losses of the past ... ... in the loss of the person you could watch ... ... But here you see yourself and are separated from yourself ... ... You think about how jealousy has led you away from yourself in recent years ... ... But you are in the land of dreams, and in the land of dreams, there are no limits for you ... ...

... ... So there must be a way through the fence ... ... Your counterpart, your second self in the land of dreams, points to a gate in the fence ... ... It is very close to you, you just hadn't seen it ... ... But now you see it ... ... You go there ... ... Above the gate hangs a sign that reads ... ... Gate of Trust ... ... And to reach yourself, you go through the open gate of trust ... ... That is the only way to yourself ... ... You walk through ... ... You walk through the gate of trust ... ... In the land of dreams, you can trust and thereby meet yourself ... ...

... ... You find yourself in the land of dreams ... ... Your path is trust ... ... Trust in the land of dreams ... ... Trust in yourself ... ... Here it is easy ... ... Here you can do everything because everything happens in your creative imagination ... ... But everything that is possible in your creative imagination is also possible in your waking life because the land of dreams is more than imagination … …

… … The land of dreams really exists … … It is pure truth … … The truth of your feelings … … You remember … … The land of dreams is deep within you … … It has always been there … … I'm just telling you about it … …

All Titles in the Series

Volume 1: Smoking Cessation
Volume 2: Anxiety and Restlessness
Volume 3: Burnout
Volume 4: Reducing Overweight
Volume 5: Coping with the Past
Volume 6: Suicidal Thoughts and Attempts
Volume 7: Psycho-Oncology
Volume 8: Obsessions and Tics
Volume 9: Self-Confidence and Decision-Making
Volume 10: Grief Work
Volume 11: Psychosomatics
Volume 12: Chronic Pain
Volume 13: Depressive Thoughts
Volume 14: Panic Attacks
Volume 15: Domestic Violence, Victim Support
Volume 16: Post-Traumatic Stress
Volume 17: Exam Anxiety and Stage Fright
Volume 18: Anti-Violence Training, Offender Support
Volume 19: Addiction Tendencies
Volume 20: Social Phobia and Fear of Contact
Volume 21: Nail Biting
Volume 22: Self-Awareness and Self-Love
Volume 23: Teeth Grinding and Night Clenching
Volume 24: Feelings of Guilt
Volume 25: Fear in Crowds
Volume 26: Fear of Flying, Aviophobia
Volume 27: Fear in Enclosed Spaces, Claustrophobia
Volume 28: Tinnitus, Ear Noises
Volume 29: Fear of Heights
Volume 30: Neurodermatitis

Volume 31: Finding Inner Balance
Volume 32: Overcoming Loneliness
Volume 33: Fear of Illness, Hypochondria
Volume 34: Anticipatory Anxiety, Fear of Fear
Volume 35: Jealousy in Relationships
Volume 36: Driving Anxiety
Volume 37: New Start after Separation
Volume 38: Fear of Injections
Volume 39: Heart Anxiety Neurosis
Volume 40: Overcoming Resentment and Anger
Volume 41: Resolving Blockages and Positive Thinking
Volume 42: Stress Reduction, Stress Management
Volume 43: Body Relaxation
Volume 44: Deep Relaxation
Volume 45: Fear of the Dark
Volume 46: Falling Asleep and Staying Asleep
Volume 47: Compulsive Buying
Volume 48: Restless Legs Syndrome
Volume 49: Bulimia
Volume 50: Anorexia
Volume 51: Overcoming Nightmares
Volume 52: Imagined Deformity
Volume 53: Overcoming Distrust, Finding Trust
Volume 54: Processing Failures
Volume 55: Humiliation, Emotional Hurt
Volume 56: Distressing Compassion, Vicarious Suffering
Volume 57: Self-Forgiveness
Volume 58: Self-Awareness, Self-Confidence
Volume 59: Saying No
Volume 60: Assertiveness
Volume 61: Setting Boundaries and Self-Assertion
Volume 62: Decision-Making Ability

Volume 63: Success Orientation
Volume 64: Ruminating, Circular Thinking
Volume 65: Accepting Pregnancy
Volume 66: Birth Preparation
Volume 67: Spiritual Opening
Volume 68: Joy of Life and Inner Lightness
Volume 69: Patience and Inner Peace
Volume 70: Fibromyalgia and Rheumatism
Volume 71: Irritable Bowel Syndrome, Crohn's Disease
Volume 72: Fear of Nausea, Emetophobia
Volume 73: Stuttering and Cluttering, Speech Flow Disorders
Volume 74: Concentration and Knowledge Anchoring
Volume 75: Vitality and Spontaneity
Volume 76: Searching for Meaning and Finding Goals
Volume 77: Life Crises, Life Events
Volume 78: Workaholism, Goal Obsession
Volume 79: Helper Syndrome, Helpless Helpers
Volume 80: Medication Abuse
Volume 81: Gambling Addiction
Volume 82: Internet Addiction, Smartphone Addiction
Volume 83: Hoarding Disorder, Compulsive Collecting
Volume 84: Conspiracy Thoughts, Overvalued Ideas
Volume 85: Fear of Operations and Treatments
Volume 86: Fear of Aging
Volume 87: Travel Anxiety
Volume 88: Anxiety When Urinating, Paruresis
Volume 89: Fear of Intimacy and Togetherness
Volume 90: Fear of Blushing
Volume 91: Coming Out in Homosexuality
Volume 92: Charisma Training
Volume 93: Migraines and Chronic Headaches
Volume 94: Overcoming Allergies, Bronchial Asthma

Volume 95: Normalizing Blood Pressure
Volume 96: Compulsive Perfectionism
Volume 97: Sports Hypnosis, Motivation
Volume 98: Sports Hypnosis, Performance Enhancement
Volume 99: Determination and Focus
Volume 100: Encountering the Inner Child
Volume 101: Cravings, Binge Eating
Volume 102: Stimulating Metabolism
Volume 103: Bipolar Mood Swings
Volume 104: Borderline, Identity Crises
Volume 105: Hypomania, Euphoria, Mania
Volume 106: Restlessness, Agitation
Volume 107: Nervous Breakdown
Volume 108: Adjustment Disorders
Volume 109: Self-Alienation, Depersonalization
Volume 110: Ending Self-Pity
Volume 111: Primary Gain of Illness
Volume 112: Secondary Gain of Illness
Volume 113: Bullying, Victim Support
Volume 114: Letting Go of Envy and Jealousy
Volume 115: Fear of Spiders, Arachnophobia
Volume 116: Fear of Dogs or Cats
Volume 117: Fear of Strangers, Xenophobia
Volume 118: Excessive Worries, Generalized Anxiety
Volume 119: Strengthening Sense of Responsibility
Volume 120: Unrequited Love, Heartache
Volume 121: Work-Life Balance
Volume 122: Letting Go of Unattainable Goals
Volume 123: Allowing and Accepting Help
Volume 124: Letting Go of Adult Children
Volume 125: Tourette Syndrome
Volume 126: Life Changes and New Starts

Volume 127: Accepting Life in a Wheelchair
Volume 128: Understanding and Overcoming Homesickness
Volume 129: Understanding and Overcoming Wanderlust
Volume 130: Dizziness, Meniere's Disease
Volume 131: Overcoming Aggression
Volume 132: Cutting and Self-Harm
Volume 133: Hair Pulling, Trichotillomania
Volume 134: Postpartum Depression
Volume 135: For Relatives of Dementia Patients
Volume 136: Self-Harm, Artificial Disorders
Volume 137: Activating Self-Healing Powers
Volume 138: Preventing Depression Relapse
Volume 139: Reactive Psychoses, Follow-Up
Volume 140: Obsessive Thoughts and Impulses
Volume 141: Compulsive Checking
Volume 142: Compulsive Counting, Symmetry Obsession
Volume 143: Compulsive Washing, Cleanliness Obsession
Volume 144: Compulsive Questioning
Volume 145: Dissociative Paralysis
Volume 146: Phantom Pain
Volume 147: Overcoming Complaining
Volume 148: Hay Fever, Pollen Allergy
Volume 149: Sexual Abuse, Victim Support
Volume 150: Standing Strong Against Sexism, #metoo
Volume 151: Binge Eating
Volume 152: Overcoming Thoughts of Revenge
Volume 153: Detachment from the Aggressor, Stockholm Syndrome
Volume 154: Courage to Separate
Volume 155: Chronic Fatigue, Exhaustion
Volume 156: Fear of the Future, Existential Anxiety
Volume 157: Excessive Worry About Children
Volume 158: Fear of Failure

Volume 159: Ending Distrust and Control
Volume 160: Dejection, Dysphoria
Volume 161: Boreout, Chronic Boredom
Volume 162: Bipolar Disorders, Relapse Prevention
Volume 163: Mania, Relapse Prevention
Volume 164: Nihilism, Feelings of Worthlessness
Volume 165: Thumb Sucking
Volume 166: Being Brave
Volume 167: Being Proud
Volume 168: Overcoming Shyness
Volume 169: Being Able to Delegate Responsibility
Volume 170: Being Able to Show Emotions
Volume 171: Letting Go of Guilt, Victim Support
Volume 172: Processing Guilt, Offender Support
Volume 173: Mood Swings, Cyclothymia
Volume 174: Lack of Drive, Vital Sadness
Volume 175: Hearing Voices with Reality Reference
Volume 176: Confident Communication
Volume 177: Standing Up for Oneself
Volume 178: Taking New Paths
Volume 179: Confident Job Application
Volume 180: No Longer Being Taken Advantage Of
Volume 181: End of Submissiveness
Volume 182: Depressive Numbness
Volume 183: Mood Drops, Affective Incontinence
Volume 184: Mood Instability
Volume 185: Somatoform Disorders
Volume 186: Stomach Ulcer, Psychosomatic
Volume 187: Accepting Amputation
Volume 188: Overcoming and Letting Go of Hatred
Volume 189: Ending Accusations
Volume 190: Allowing Tears, Being Able to Cry

Volume 191: Finding and Sorting Repressed Feelings
Volume 192: Somatoform Pain
Volume 193: Living Autonomously
Volume 194: Anhedonia, Joylessness
Volume 195: Persistent Sadness
Volume 196: Obesity, Food Addiction
Volume 197: Parents of Abused Children
Volume 198: Letting Go and Letting Be
Volume 199: Childhood Sexual Abuse
Volume 200: Fear of Loss

www.ingramcontent.com/pod-product-compliance
Lightning Source LLC
Chambersburg PA
CBHW030509220526
45464CB00006B/2717